LSD: The Truth About Acid

The Ultimate Beginner's Guide to Lysergic Acid Diethylamide and Its Full Effects

I0503182

Table Of Contents

Introduction

You've probably heard about "LSD" or "Acid" some time before. Maybe you've heard about how consuming it is supposed to give a person some semblance of euphoria and even alter one's way of thinking. So, what exactly is LSD and what does it do?

This short and concise book will focus on the history of this incredible tool, the science behind it, and how consuming it can affect one's body. Most practically, we will also look at the pros and cons of this tool and how it compares to other similar "drugs".

In this book we are aiming to look at this topic in an unbiased light. We are not promoting the consumption of LSD or similar drugs, per se, but we want to make sure that if someone is interested in this controversial topic, he or she can reach more informed conclusions.

We hope that you are able to learn a thing or two!

Chapter 1:

What is LSD?

Overview

LSD, or lysergic acid diethylamide, is a psychedelic drug of the ergoline family. It is used as either an entheogen or a recreational drug. Ergoline is a chemical compound whose derivatives are largely used for the purpose of vasoconstriction. Ergoline alkaloids produce psychedelic effects, and ergoline is the active ingredient in LSD.

As an entheogen, LSD is ingested to put the user in a meditative state of consciousness for spiritual purposes. As a recreational drug, however, LSD is considered one of the most potent hallucinogenic chemicals known to man. LSD typically alters the user's mood and causes him or her to see, hear, and feel things that may seem tangible, but in reality, they do not exist.

Although LSD does not put users at a risk for dependency, it produces extremely strong psychological effects. The most common effects of LSD are an altered mood and sense of time, altered thinking processes, both closed-eye visuals and open-eyed visuals, and synesthesia. Adverse reactions to LSD have also been documented, including paranoia and anxiety.

LSD is manufactured from lysergic acid found in ergot—a fungus that grows on grains. Typically, LSD is produced in crystal form within illegal and clandestine laboratories. Upon distribution, LSD is converted from its crystal form to its liquid form. Pure LSD is tasteless, colorless, and odorless in either form.

Uses

Medical

Currently, LSD has no recognized medical value or use. This is largely due to the fact that LSD does not benefit a person's health nor physical or mental well-being, at least not yet shown by the research.

Spiritual

Some cultures consider LSD an entheogen, so they use the drug for spiritual purposes. An entheogen is a substance that, when ingested, produces a spiritual experience. LSD has been documented to cause a user to experience lucid sensations and intense spiritual occurrences, during which users claim they have come into contact with a spiritual order.

It is suggested that ancient civilizations used a rudimentary form of LSD during rituals and other spiritual practices in order to feel closer to the gods.

Recreational

LSD is classified as an illegal drug worldwide. As such, it is a controlled substance whose manufacturing is also illegal. Nevertheless, LSD is commonly used around the world as a recreational drug. Users often find enjoyment in the drug's psychedelic and hallucinogenic effects, especially when combined with artistic experiences, such as music or movies.

Pharmacokinetics

The effects of LSD generally wear off anywhere between 6 to 12 hours following consumption. The duration and intensity of its effects depend on the dosage, as well as the user's weight and tolerance. As long as significant levels of LSD are present in the blood, the drug's effects will continue.

Physical Properties

The salts that LSD contains are triboluminescent, meaning they emit flashes of white light when shaken. As a whole, LSD is fluorescent, and the drug glows bluish-white under a black light.

Synthesis

LSD synthesis involves reacting diethylamine with an activated form of lysergic acid. Lysergic acid is made through hydrolysis of lysergamides and ergoline alkaloids known as ergotamine. However, ergotamine is no longer an essential component of

LSD because the drug can now be produced synthetically.

Dosage

LSD dosages are very low, usually coming in micrograms, or millionths of a gram. In comparison, other recreational drugs are usually measured in thousandths of a gram. One dose of LSD can be anywhere between 40 and 500 micrograms, which is equivalent to one-tenth of the mass of a grain of sand. An average user can feel noticeable effects and have vivid hallucinations with just 25 micrograms of LSD.

Because of its low dosage requirements, it is almost impossible for a person to overdose on LSD. The lethal dose is 200 micrograms per one kilogram of body weight. This means that a lethal dose for a person weighing 180 pounds is 16,000 micrograms.

Legal Status

The United Nations Convention requires its parties to prohibit LSD. Medical and scientific research centered on LSD in humans, however, is legal.

In the United States, LSD is a controlled substance classified under Schedule I of the Controlled Substances Act of 1970. As a Schedule I drug, LSD is illegal to distribute, possess, process, or manufacture in the Untied States. Being classified as a Schedule I drug signifies that LSD meets three criteria:

It has a high potential for abuse.

It has no legitimate medical use.

There is a lack of safety for its use.

Production

Because LSD is active in such small doses, it allows numerous doses to be synthesized from just a small amount of raw material. Just 25 kilograms of raw material can produce 5 kilograms of pure LSD in crystal form, which is equivalent to approximately 100 million doses. In addition, because the dosages are so minuscule, it is relatively easy to smuggle them past country borders.

Laboratory equipment is used in the manufacturing of LSD. Producers and chemists must have a strong working knowledge of the field of organic chemistry. It only takes a couple days to produce 100 grams of LSD. LSD is not normally mass-produced, and it is usually produced in small batches.

Distribution

Before LSD is distributed, it is first converted from a crystal to a liquid. Liquid solutions are then either distributed in small vials or allowed to soak into a distribution medium. LSD can be sold on the streets in tablet form known as microdots, on sugar cubes, or as gelatin squares called "windowpanes." Depending on the mode of distribution, LSD can either be swallowed or absorbed by holding it under the tongue.

LSD is more commonly sold as a thin sheet of blotter paper, also called "computer acid" due to its resemblance to a computer chip. These blotter papers are made via soaking a larger sheet of blotter paper in a solution of LSD, alcohol, and water. The blotter paper is then cut into small squares, and one square of blotter paper equals one dose of LSD. This blotter paper is usually printed with designs like swirls or spirals before soaking.

LSD in Popular Culture

Since becoming popularized in the United States by Timothy Leary, a proclaimed "LSD-guru," many notorious figures became associated with this intriguing drug. Lewis Carroll, the author of *Alice in Wonderland*, was said to be under the influence of

LSD, or a similar psychedelic of the same class, when he wrote his famous book.

The 1960s was considered the Psychedelic Era due to the influence of LSD and "magic mushrooms" in popular culture. The members of The Beatles openly used LSD, which was obvious in the lyrics of some of their hit songs (most notable of all is "Lucy in the Sky with Diamonds"). Jefferson Airplane, Jimi Hendrix, Pink Floyd, and other popular bands of the '60s and '70s used LSD frequently and openly.

Chapter 2:

History of LSD

Albert Hoffman, a Swiss chemist, synthesized LSD for the first time in 1938. What he originally wanted to formulate was a blood stimulant, not a recreational drug. At the time of LSD synthesis, Hoffman was not aware of the drug's hallucinogenic effects. In 1943, however, Hoffman ingested samples of LSD by accident and found that the drug did indeed possess psychedelic properties, which produced extremely vivid hallucinations.

In 1947, Sandoz Pharmaceutical, the company Albert Hoffman worked for, introduced LSD as a psychiatric drug. After testing the drug on animals, the pharmaceutical company began supplying researchers and psychiatrists with free samples of LSD. Studies and experiments were conducted in an attempt to determine any medical value that LSD might have.

In the 1950s, the CIA began researching the prospect of LSD as a chemical weapon. The research program was code named "Project MKULTRA." Experiments conducted by the agency involved the distribution of LSD to doctors, military personnel, mentally ill patients, and even CIA employees. The CIA then studied the reactions of the test subjects to the drug. The experiments were usually conducted without the knowledge of the test subjects in order to reach definitive conclusions.

The CIA noted that LSD was capable of rendering an entire group of people—even whole military forces—indifferent to their surroundings and unresponsive to their situations. According to their conclusions, LSD interfered with judgment and thought processes, and the drug even created confusion and fear in those who ingested it.

Prominent individuals began advocating LSD consumption in the 1960s. American psychologist, Timothy Leary, is quoted as encouraging his students to "turn on, tune in, and drop out." Out of this support for LSD rose a counterculture of drug use. Before the end of the '60s, LSD use had spread all throughout the United States, eventually reaching the shores of Europe. In 1967, the United States banned the drug and made LSD possession illegal. Legal psychiatric use of LSD continued in Switzerland until 1993.

During the 1980s, LSD use saw a decline before skyrocketing again in the '90s. In the early 2000s, LSD was commonly used among young adults at raves and other all-night dance clubs, in particular.

Chapter 3:

The Science Behind LSD

One of the most distinguishing aspects of LSD is its capability to produce hallucinations in users. Test subjects of mind control experiments conducted decades ago reported seeing walls melt, eyes falling down faces like tears, feeling spiders scurrying all over their bodies, and cracks appearing on people's faces while under the influence of LSD.

Hallucinations occur because LSD imitates serotonin—a chemical messenger, or neurotransmitter, in the brain. Some researchers refer to serotonin as a "feel-good" chemical. Serotonin positively affects mood, social behavior, sleep, and sexual desire. Among experts, it is believed that serotonin deficiency is a common cause of depression. Additionally, some researchers suspect that serotonin is responsible for helping humans keep a handle on perception by preventing hallucinations.

LSD targets one of fourteen different serotonin receptors in the brain. This specific serotonin receptor is called 5-HT2A. When LSD targets 5-HT2A, it throws senses into overdrive and can cause confusion. This results in seeing vivid images that are completely uncharacteristic of a person's sense of perception. These images, or hallucinations, usually fool the brain into believing that they are real.

Most LSD effects occur in the region of the brain responsible for regulating cognition, mood, and perception. This area of the brain is called the prefrontal cortex, and it is sometimes referred to as "the seal of good judgment." The prefrontal cortex also controls impulses and intense emotions.

In a sober person, the brain processes information "correctly." It starts in the thalamus, which is located on top of the brain stem. The thalamus is the part of the brain where sensory perceptions are directed. When the thalamus receives information, it acts as a gatekeeper that decides what is relevant and irrelevant. It also routes the information to the proper location of the body.

In a person under the influence of LSD, however, the thalamus does not process information "correctly," so LSD inhibits the proper function of the thalamus. When a person is on LSD so is the "gatekeeper." This allows the passage of unprocessed information into the consciousness. Before long, walls begin to warp and colors seem much brighter than normal.

Chapter 4:

The Effects of LSD

Effects typically begin roughly 20 minutes after ingestion. When a user begins to feel a tingling sensation throughout his or her body, it is a clear sign that the drug has reached the user's bloodstream. About an hour after this initial effect, the effects tend to reach their peak. It is during this time that a user's pupils begin to dilate as the body temperature rises and the heart rate speeds up. The peak can last for a couple of hours, during which hallucinations may begin. Colors may appear more vibrant and sounds may seem richer. Users may notice tiny details that they've never noticed before.

The trip gradually wears off, usually leaving the user feeling drained of energy. LSD psychologically affects the user, leaving him or her with the memories of either a good or bad trip. The memories and after-effects remain, but they tend to fade over time unless documented.

The effects of LSD range from mild to intense. Effects may be physical, psychological, or sensory. Numerous side effects—both pleasant and unpleasant—of LSD have been known to occur.

One common effect among many LSD users is what they call a "bad trip." A bad trip is when a trip goes wrong, per se. Users who have experienced a bad trip say it is similar to a living hell.

Physical Effects

Physical reactions to LSD will vary and can be nonspecific. Some common physical effects include the following:

Reduced Appetite

Because of this symptom, LSD can actually inspire weight loss. Most of the weight lost while under the influence of LSD is typically water weight.

Sleeplessness

Frequent hallucinations can keep a user up at night, especially if these hallucinations are frightening.

Pupil Dilation

Psychedelics tend to cause pupil dilation because they block certain receptors in the brain responsible for pupil constriction. When the pupils are no longer capable of constriction, it results in dilation.

Cottonmouth

This is a condition characterized by dryness in the mouth. LSD affects the function of salivary glands, which results in dryness of the mouth.

Numbness

Users often report a tingling feeling or a loss of sensation in their fingers and toes during an LSD trip. This sensation is often accompanied with an uncharacteristic coldness of the fingers and/or toes.

Nausea

Feeling nauseous as the trip nears its peak is common, particularly if the user is tripping on a full stomach.

Hypothermia/Hyperthermia

Both conditions are known effects of LSD. However, they are typically associated with LSD overdose.

Increased Body Temperature

Hallucinogens tend to interfere with a user's body temperature. This phenomenon is known as drug-induced fever, or drug-induced hyperthermia.

Goosebumps

LSD-induced chills are not uncommon. Users call the phenomenon "acid chills."

Perspiration

Some LSD users tend to sweat profusely while using the drug. This may be due to the increased body temperature that accompanies a trip, as well as nervousness in some users.

Increased Blood Pressure

LSD raises blood pressure and there is no way around it. The higher the dose of LSD, the higher a user's blood pressure rises in response.

Elevated Heart Rate

Increased heart rate during LSD use can either be a small or large. Sometimes an increased heart rate during a trip can lead to a bad trip, especially if the user is in poor health.

Psychological Effects

Psychological side effects of LSD use also varies, but here are the most frequently reported mental effects:

Hallucinations

As one of the most powerful hallucinogenic drugs in the world, this effect is the most common from LSD use. A hallucination is a phenomenon that plays with one's senses. While some hallucinations may be pleasant to the senses and visually appealing, other hallucinations can be frightening, which is the gist of bad trips. When a user is deeply rooted in his or her hallucination, the user may lose their grip on reality. This is why a sober partner is a necessity for a less experienced user.

Delusions

When the user has a delusion during an LSD trip, he or she strongly believes in a certain thing that is not true, even if that particular thing is physically impossible. The user's beliefs during an episode of delusion are unyielding, even when presented with proof that verifies the impossibility of the beliefs. One may believe that he is the king or that she has been brainwashed by extraterrestrials. These delusions may even lead to paranoia.

Perceptual Distortions

Distortion of the senses is a common psychological effect of LSD. The user may have an impaired sense of time, where six hours feels like one. Colors and shapes may seem distorted as well.

Anxiety

During a trip, the user may feel exceptionally anxious about nothing in particular. Anxiety is the body's response to danger or a potential threat. Anxiety can become evident through physical manifestations, such as tremors and increased heart rate.

HPPD

This is an acronym for Hallucinogen Persisting Perception Disorder. HPPD is a phenomenon that mainly occurs after a trip is over. It is an altered perception that one is experiencing an LSD trip even when he or she is not. HPPD is a possible outcome, especially while the drug is still running through the user's bloodstream. Uncontrollable flashbacks may occur, rendering the user incompetent by preventing him or her from functioning as they normally would under sober circumstances.

Synesthesia

Synesthesia is a condition in which the sense impression relating to one sense or part of the body is produced by stimulation of another sense or part of the body. It is an abnormal blending of the senses that can be caused by LSD use. People with synesthesia may see sounds or taste words. They may even feel a sensation on their skin when they listen to music or when they smell certain scents. This is often why LSD users have trouble explaining their trip to those who have never ingested LSD.

Psychosis

Psychosis is a severe mental condition that may accompany LSD use, though only temporary. People with psychosis have thoughts and emotions that are so impaired that all contact with reality is lost. Like a delusional state, psychotics have a distorted sense of reality.

Psychological Dependence

This is a form of dependence that involves emotional withdrawal symptoms upon cessation of drug use. While it is not possible to become addicted to LSD it is possible to develop a tolerance for the drug. People who have developed a high tolerance for LSD need higher doses of the drug to achieve the same effect. When a user becomes psychologically dependent on LSD, he or she may feel compelled to continue using the drug for no definitive reason.

Suicidal Thoughts

LSD is among the recreational drugs that may lead to suicide. Other drugs with the same effect include PCP and cocaine. Suicidal thoughts may be a result of LSD-related illnesses, such as depression and sleep deprivation.

Long Term Effects of LSD Use

While the initial effects of LSD wear off after a day, the drug may cause long-term effects that may have a lifelong negative impact on the user. The long-term effects of LSD use may vary depending on the user's drug habits, but these effects are likely to become serious. As such, heavy LSD users have an increased risk of experiencing long-term effects.

Long-term effects include:

Mood swings

Lack of motivation

Damaged vision

Flashbacks, or HPPD

Tolerance, which can lead to fatal drug overdose

Mental impairment, or a reduced ability to reason and think rationally

Inability to communicate properly

Suicidal thoughts

Depression

Anxiety

Schizophrenia

Psychosis

Difficulty recognizing reality

Panic attacks

LSD users may also experience indirect consequences as a result of drug use, including:

Relationship problems with friends and family

Lack of skills to cope with the challenges of daily life

STDs due to unprotected sex

Criminal charges as a result of actions while under the influence of LSD

Sexual assault

Lack of success in work or school

Pregnancy complications

Treatment is possible for long-term LSD effects. Because LSD is not physically addictive, rehab is not an option. However, there are treatment methods available to those who are psychologically addicted to the drug. A user may need therapy in addition to a solid support system if he or she develops psychosis or depression. There is no cure, however, for the other long-term effects of LSD, such as acid flashbacks.

Health Risks of LSD Use

Every trip is different, and the effects are often unpredictable. It all depends on the dosage, the quality of the drug, the company kept and setting, and the user's personality. There is no way of knowing whether one will have a good trip or a bad one. However, there are a few steps to proactively create a buffer for one's trip, including being in the company of trusted friends, being in a safe, controlled environment, clearing one's mind of emotional baggage, and ensuring the quality of the LSD is top-notch.

Some users may experience extreme mood swings and paranoia. The worst part is that they often cannot distinguish between reality and the sensations created by LSD. Other users may experience terrifying delusions and hallucinations that they cannot escape from. Fear of death, insanity, and losing control is common during a trip. Large doses of LSD tend to alter a user's personality to the point where he or she is no longer recognized. The world becomes distorted to the user, and his or her sense of self may change for the worst. The user's ability to think and rationalize becomes impaired, and what seems a harmless pursuit may end in death or arrest.

Frequent LSD use can result in disassociation and a lack of interest in the things that one once enjoyed. Sometimes relationships are jeopardized, as is the user's life. This is possible if depression is a factor. When LSD is used during pregnancy, LSD causes uterine contractions, which are extremely dangerous for the fetus.

Sometimes, quitting LSD cold turkey is not enough to avoid health risks. The drug's long-term effects may stay for the rest of one's life. LSD-induced psychosis may even be impossible to recover from, even with therapy.

Chapter 5:

Pros and Cons of LSD

Just because LSD and other psychedelics are taboo and have bad reputations by the popular media doesn't mean they are completely bad. Surprisingly, LSD has a few notable pros to combat its cons.

Pros of LSD

There's no denying it: tripping is fun, provided the user is having a good trip. Colors are brighter and senses are more enhanced. Some hallucinations may even be pleasant.

LSD is relatively cheap in comparison to other recreational drugs. Some users pay only $5 per dose, and some have even claimed to trip for free. Buying LSD wholesale is also cheap by comparison.

LSD is actually the safest of the recreational psychedelic drugs. It takes you to your peak, and then brings you down with a feeling of well-being. At the end of the "comedown" LSD makes you feel cleansed, albeit pretty drained.

LSD cannot be used repeatedly due to tolerance. One week is all it takes for the drug's full effects to return in most users.

LSD has the lowest risk for dependency out of all the recreational psychedelic drugs out there.

Euphoria is another positive aspect of LSD. The psychedelic effects of the drug make the user happy, bringing out a smile that acid users call "the psychedelic grin."

Because of the heightened senses that come with a trip, LSD makes sexual intercourse much more pleasurable. Sex drive tends to be higher during a trip, and sexual performance is often significantly better.

LSD tends to bring about creativity. This is because the drug stimulates the brain into overdrive. There is no doubt that some of the greatest musical and cinematic pieces were inspired by psychedelic use. Because of this, artists often view LSD as a tool to help them express their creative thoughts.

LSD does not cause any neurological damage, nor does it cause chronic physiological damage.

Death from LSD use is extremely rare.

LSD is nontoxic.

LSD increases awareness, attention to detail, and energy.

Cons of LSD

Bad trips. They can be traumatizing, especially when it is relived in the occurrence of a flashback. Also, bad trips can last for 10 to 12 hours in the worst case.

Overdose is possible, especially when the user has developed a tolerance for LSD, which would cause him or her to take a higher dose of the drug than is safe.

Nausea comes with the territory, and it can last throughout the entirety of a trip.

It is nearly impossible to hide the fact that you are under the influence of LSD for a less experienced user. Dilated pupils, redness in the eyes, and profuse sweating are dead giveaways if one is around sharp and sober people.

LSD is illegal. In the United States, the possession, production, purchase, and sale of LSD can get you fined and/or thrown in jail.

Paranoia often accompanies any hallucinogen, and it can ruin the LSD experience if it gets out of control.

LSD can cause jaw tension and even lockjaw, which is reported to be extremely uncomfortable.

Megalomania has been known to occur in some users, which can lead to humiliation. Megalomania is the condition of being obsessed with the exercise of power.

Chapter 6:

LSD Compared to Other Recreational Drugs

LSD is an extremely unique recreational drug. It is a hallucinogen and psychedelic at the same time. There are many aspects and factors that set LSD apart from other recreational drugs.

LSD vs. Marijuana

LSD ergot and marijuana are both products of nature. Both of the drugs are hallucinogens, both are mind-altering, and both have the effect of opening the mind. However, that is where the similarities of these two drugs end.

The LSD high and the marijuana high are significantly different. While LSD is a cerebral experience, marijuana is more centered on the body. LSD acts as a stimulant while marijuana acts as a sedative. In terms of mental effects, LSD is much more intense than marijuana (under relatively moderate doses). The average user still has the ability to function in public while under the influence of marijuana, but LSD can take away all ability to function for some individuals.

LSD vs. Ecstasy

Both LSD and ecstasy can be sold in pill form. Sometimes, ecstasy is dipped in an LSD solution, thereby combining the effects of both drugs. Ecstasy, however, is not classified as a hallucinogen, but it can contain traces of hallucinogens depending on how it is formulated. Each drug has been used in psychological warfare experiments, both drugs are globally outlawed, and both loosen inhibition. Both of them also make one sensitive to light, experience fluid loss, and causes jaw tension.

LSD and ecstasy are two different chemicals that produce completely different effects. LSD is like a mind high, while ecstasy is a body high. Ecstasy plays on the hormones, and LSD does not. The comedown on ecstasy is grim, but the comedown on LSD promotes a feeling of well-being.

LSD vs. PCP

LSD and PCP share almost no similarities. They are both recreational drugs, and that is about it. LSD is a psychedelic drug, while PCP is a dissociative anesthetic. LSD enhances alertness and causes sleeplessness, and PCP makes a user feel relaxed and drowsy. LSD diminishes the user's sense of self, but PCP enhances the user's ego. LSD gives the effect of synesthesia and colorful visuals, however PCP detaches the user's mind from his or her body.

LSD vs. Psychedelic Mushrooms

LSD and "shrooms" are both drugs that produce psychedelic effects. They are both derived from fungus, and they are both tryptamine substances. Both psychedelics can also cause bad trips.

The mushroom experience is significantly different compared to the LSD experience. The LSD high is more colorful and vibrant while the mushroom high is more nature-oriented. The effects of LSD last roughly 12 hours, while the mushroom effects last only six.

LSD produces a lesser degree of anxiety than mushrooms. The LSD high is less incapacitating than mushrooms. Mushroom users tend to be more of a couch potato while LSD users can be more like social butterflies. LSD only requires a small dose to produce hallucinations, and mushrooms require a larger dose to produce the same effect.

LSD vs. Cocaine

LSD and cocaine are both popular choices for recreational use. Each drug could result in suicidal thoughts, both are stimulants, and they both make the user social and talkative. LSD, however, is cheaper in cost than cocaine. The LSD high is significantly longer than cocaine as well. Also, LSD is much safer than cocaine. It is nearly impossible to die from an LSD overdose, but a cocaine overdose is likely to kill you. LSD is not addictive, but cocaine, however, is. LSD does not necessarily produce organ damage, but cocaine can damage the heart and nose.

LSD vs. Heroin

LSD and heroin are two very different drugs. LSD is almost impossible to overdose on, but it is relatively easy to overdose on heroin. Long-term heroin use can cause irreversible damage and diseases like tuberculosis and pneumonia, and long-term LSD use, by comparison, does not cause any lung-related health conditions. Heroin use cessation causes extreme withdrawal symptoms, and LSD cessation does not. Heroin is highly addictive, but LSD is not addictive at all.

LSD vs. Amphetamines

Amphetamines are recreational drugs that may be referred to as "speed." Both LSD and speed are stimulants, thus they both give the user energy. Both drugs also tend to make the user anxious, overactive, and jittery, and they both also cause temporary psychosis. LSD, however, is a relatively safer chemical than amphetamines. While LSD is typically sold as microdots or blotter papers, speed is sold as a powder that can be snorted or rubbed into the gums. The street price of LSD is cheaper than the price of speed.

Chapter 7:

The Future of LSD

LSD is currently used as a research tool. Studies are being conducted on LSD's potential healing power. The drug serves as a means to revive neuroscience and is used in studies about the serotonin receptors in the brain. LSD is a drug that acts as a stimulant, and therefore it may be used to treat migraines and cancer in the future. The psychedelic could quite possibly effectively treat anxiety, depression, and obsessive-compulsive disorder.

Potential Medical Uses of LSD

Because LSD has been used for decades in psychiatry, the drug does not have as bad of a reputation as others in its class. Some researchers believe that LSD has the potential for therapeutic use. The following are some potential therapeutic uses of lysergic acid diethylamide:

Pain

Studies have shown that LSD is just as effective in treating pain as traditional opiates. LSD has the potential of acting as a painkiller for both chronic and acute pain caused by trauma or cancer. The drug's pain-relieving effects have a longer duration than conventional analgesics.

Alcoholism

In the 1950s, experiments were conducted to determine if LSD was an effective treatment for alcoholism. The success rate was a little over 50%.

Psychotherapy

LSD can uncover repressed memories, so it is currently being studied for psychotherapeutic use.

Creativity Enhancement

While creativity enhancement is not technically a medical use, it is a positive way to use LSD. LSD and other psychedelics may be useful for those working on a creative project, as the drug enables one to see and think without one's usual defenses.

Legalization

The truth is that LSD as a recreational drug is no closer to legalization than it was 50 years ago. While the future of LSD therapy is promising, the worldwide ban of the drug as a recreational drug is not likely to be lifted. LSD may, however, become legalized for therapeutic use in the future, with new laws and guidelines that will govern the possession and use of the drug.

There is currently no movement underway that supports the recreational legalization of LSD. Recreational legalization of LSD would lead to a shift in society. LSD will likely remain a Class A drug for years to come (Class A drugs are considered to be the most harmful drugs).

Conclusion

Thank you for reading this! We hope this short, concise book was able to teach you a thing or two about the intriguing LSD tool.

Whatever you call LSD—acid, California Sunshine, Electric Kool-Aid—its effects are all the same, and it's not a surprise that LSD is popular. It's extremely easy to take, doesn't involve any pipes or paraphernalia, and just a tiny amount is all you need to feel its full effects. Furthermore, LSD is easy to conceal and not so easy to detect. Also, it's relatively safe compared to other recreational drugs.

Nevertheless, LSD can be dangerous in the long run, as long-term use is usually accompanied with severe health risks. Like with all drugs, LSD must be used with caution. It is possible to escape dependence on the drug with the proper help and a solid support system. Remember that there is always a way out.

Now that you understand the important factors regarding LSD, you can decide if you want to try it, or if you can inform your friends who ask you about it. Plus, a little addition to your knowledge doesn't hurt, right? Our world is becoming increasingly interested in the use of LSD and other out-of-body experience inducing substances, in hopes to enhance the human experience on Earth.

If you've learned anything from this book, please take the time to share your thoughts by sending me a personal message, or even posting a review on Amazon. It would be greatly appreciated and I try my best to get back to every message!

Thank you and good luck in your journey!

www.ingramcontent.com/pod-product-compliance
Lightning Source LLC
Chambersburg PA
CBHW070847180526
45168CB00002B/989